Affirmations For Coping With Infertility

To help you manage stress, anxiety, sadness and
other emotions, so you can find balance
and rediscover yourself

Andreia Trigo

© 2017 Andreia Trigo
All rights reserved.
ISBN 10: 1977874266
ISBN 13: 978-1977874269

This book is dedicated to my dear family and partner,
who have offered me their unyielding support,
helped me mourn the losses and ultimately
rise above the challenges of infertility.

*

Each (in)fertility journey is unique and challenging in its own way. Facing such a diagnosis and envisioning a life of involuntary childlessness is daunting, triggers different emotions, such as shock, denial, anger, resentment, stress, anxiety, sadness. It's a wound that never heals and forever hurts.

There's times of inevitable and unbearable suffering when getting on with other aspects of life seems too difficult. But as challenging as it may be, life does go on, and slowly we need to find ways of living meaningfully.

Affirmations are a way of managing those emotions, finding balance, building strength and rediscovering yourself.

What is an affirmation?

An affirmation is a declaration or a strong statement of something that is true. When repeated daily, over time, the intention of the positive outcome becomes an internalised belief. When we believe without a doubt that something is true, we are increasing the likelihood of what we want to manifest actually happening.

The way you think about yourself, your body, and your (in)fertility journey have an impact on you, on your relationship with yourself and with others who are meaningful to you.

So, next time you feel stress or any other negative emotion, take a deep breath and read an affirmation out loud. Repeat it 3 times. Allow it to enter your mind, body and soul and become part of you.

Some of the affirmations in this book might resonate with you more than others. Choose the ones that are meaningful to you.

This journey is making you incredibly strong and resilient!

Andreia Trigo

*

I now release anything that is holding me back from coping with infertility.

I take care of myself, my body and my mind.

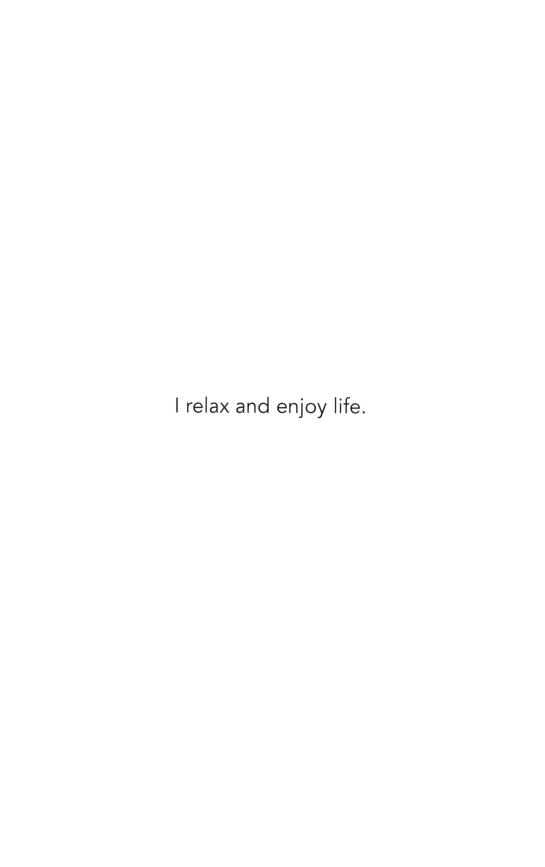

I release fears about my worth and womanhood.

I trust that everything happens in the right timing, and for a higher purpose.

I trust my body.

I have everything it takes to live a meaningful life.

I allow myself to be loved, and to create a new life out of that love.

I willingly release old thinking patterns based on fear and self-doubt. I allow new ones based on love and self-confidence.

I allow new beginnings in my life.

Good things are going to happen.

I accept the gift of life and joy.

I trust that the universe gives me exactly what I need at exactly the right time. Everything works out perfectly.

I now release all unwanted built-up emotional patterns that prevent me from connecting to my inner self.

My courage is stronger
Than my fear.

Everything I feel and experience is part of the great lesson of growing to be the best human being I can be.

I am grateful to be alive and healthy.

I am in perfect health.
My body is perfect.

My choices are based on facts
not fear.

I now choose to create peace within me and around me.

How I feel matters and I choose to feel safe.

I choose to believe good things about myself, my body and my mind.

I trust my body.

New balance is coming to my body.
My body is beautiful just the
way it is.

I am calm and centered when looking forward to finding a balanced life.

I accept the help of others with an open heart and mind.

I have the confidence to ask for help and receive help when I need it.

I am listening to my body and its needs.

I choose to see the beauty in this whole process of becoming stronger.

I am calm, cool and confident.

There may be difficult days but I am strong, determined and resilient.

Breathing in, I know I am a great woman. Breathing out, I AM a great woman.

I am totally relaxed and at ease.

I am becoming more and more confident about my ability to live a meaningful life.

My sadness lifts away and renewed sense of hope settles in my heart.

I will not obsess over things that are out of my control.

I trust and love myself.

I am too positive to be doubtful, too optimistic to be fearful, and too determined to be defeated.

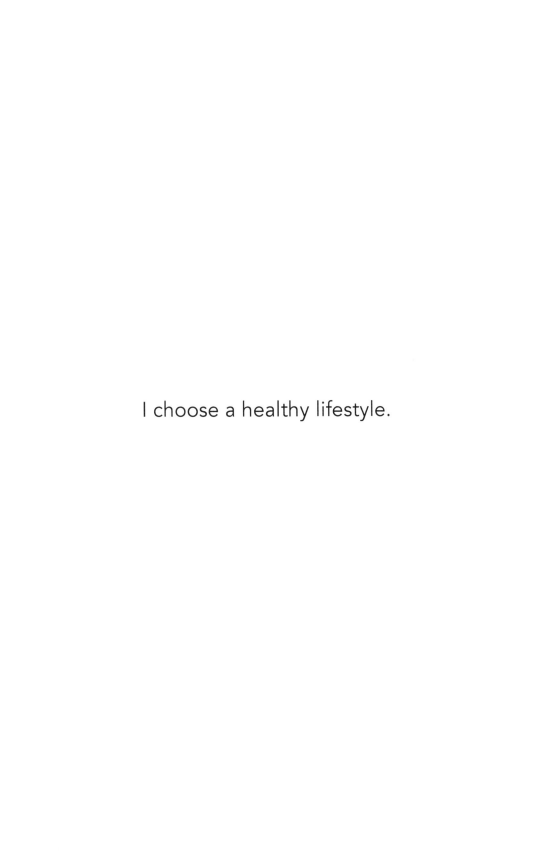

I choose healthy foods every day. I now crave only foods that increase my wellbeing.

I easily avoid hydrogenated, highly processed foods and I enjoy simple foods made by nature.

I take care of myself.

I am absolutely committed to creating a happy home and environment for myself.

I am a great woman.
My partner is lucky to have me.

I walk into every situation expecting the best.

I now choose positive thoughts that nurture and support my life.

Nothing is important enough
to stress me.

I am loving and thankful toward my partner.

I am surrounded by love.

I am worthy of love and have the capacity to love.

I have an amazing support system.

I commit to a permanent state of peace, love, joy and gratitude.

I commit to opening my mind to more useful ways of thinking.

I create the life I want.

I am grateful and love my body, just the way it is, and because of the way it is.

I get fulfillment from being my true self.

I trust everything is evolving the way it is supposed to.

I am thankful for my struggle because without it, I wouldn't have stumbled across my strength.

I surrender to what is, let go of what was and have faith in what will be.